10 X's BETTER
The Greater Offer

By:
Shakinah Glory Russell PhD

Unless otherwise indicated, all scriptures quotations are taken from the N.I.V-ESV-NASB- AMP-NEB or KJV of the Bible.

10 X's Better
The Greater Offer
ISBN- ISBN-13: 978-1503374171
Copyright © 2015 : Shakinah Glory Russell
Printed in the United States of America

Acknowledgements

Dr. Joel Wallach for saving my children's & my life, we were vitamin & mineral deficient and now were not only taking 90 to life supplements I'm a C.E.O of your foundation and is pattering my life after you traveling and teaching the importance of health in nutrition along with the word of God Thank You ;-).

D.R.O Florida Apostle Erica & Raymond Austin Thank you for your diligence in unfailing love in the Ministry God bless you.

Dr. William Morse, Pastor Richard & Andrea Ledford of Tallahassee Florida, Thank You for your perpetual encouragement. **Shakinah's; Touch** out **R**each **M**inistries (S.T.O.R.M) Love you & God bless.

To My husband Apostle: Joseph R. Russell, Kevin, Se'Quoya, Miracle, Ruth & Benjamin for your undying love and support.

As always saving the best for last, My Heart-soul, my mind & my inspiration (1) for the My Father (1) for His Son the only begotten & (1) for the HOLY GHOST!!! , In Jesus Name.

Contents

1. Predestined Preparation 1

2. Essential Minerals for Maintenance & Recover............... 14

3. Essential Vitamins for Maintenance & Recovery............23

4. Type I& typeII Diabetes 24

5. High Blood Pressure Healing...............................34

6. Ear, Teeth Health..38

7. Ear Health……………………………….……..40

8. Cholesterol...41

9. Kidney Health …….…….......……… ………………..43

10 Finding Good Ground …………..………………….45

11 Winning the war in your body ……..………………47

12 How to Naturally Low Stomach Acid………………..…50

13 Emotional Healing …………………………………51

14 The Missing Link (Which Mineral are you Missing?…..…..55

15 Fibroid Tumors drive out …………. …...………....56

Which foods give the best nutrition?

Predestined Preparation

When God created the heavens, earth, herbs, plants, and animals he made us interchangeably – interdependent.
Many years of research and autopsies have been completed to help us understand sickness, caused by disease, and finally death.
Different animals act as a model for the study of human illness. For example: Rabbits suffer from <u>Atherosclerosis</u> (Harding of the arteries). As well as <u>emphysema</u> and Birth Defects such as <u>Spinal Bifida</u>.
Dogs suffer from <u>Cancer</u>, <u>Diabetes</u>, <u>Cataracts</u>, <u>Ulcers</u> and Bleeding Disorders such as <u>Hemophilia.</u>
Our parallel makeup makes them natural candidates for research into all of these disorders.
This is a reflection of our God: Jehovah Elohim creator of everything.
The nutritional elements required to maximize our life span is **25-50** years longer, being human and having vertebrae; (the series of small bones forming the backbone) <u>like a bird</u> consists of **60** minerals, **16** vitamins, **12** amino acids, & **2** fatty acids. You can trace all illness, chronic and otherwise, result of a person deficient in one or more mineral.
Did you know that we've eliminated more than 1,000 diseases in animals including birth defects that still plague human beings today?
Dog, cat, chicken, monkey, & rat food have all the essential nutrients that are required for quality health and a maximized life span; even the dumbest animals have the perfect diet.
Baby food only has **13** minerals, what happened to the other **47**?

Our children only get 20% of what they need to have all the essential nutrients that are required for quality health and maximized life span. Human beings are supposed to be at the top of the food chain. "Why are we at the bottom"?

This act is irresponsible & neglectful to deliberately prescribe the amount of vitamins & minerals to ensure that one day children will become ill, our children are left open like a piece of sliced meat. They are deprived of having a 100% nutritional diet. Children need a specific amount of vitamins, minerals and fatty acids to have a complete diet; one that will ensure that they will grow to be healthy individuals that lead healthy lives. The system sends people to jail for the mistreatment of children. What about this? Isn't nutrition the fundamentals for starting and maintaining a healthy lifestyle?

Our children are already exposed to violence, racism, and ill spoken words, we totally get that! But, nutrition is overlooked big time and it has been the silent killer of millions of people for more than a decade.

We must understand that Doctors don't have to give us a cure even if one is available, so they don't; many will just medicate you until you die. Doctor- A person who is qualified to treat people who are ill/verses Healer- One that heals or attempts to heal, especially a faith healer. Doctors treat symptoms not heal.

It's like the video games where the dragon has taken the keys and have locked away you're healing and you have to chase him down to get your stuff back. When you find him in the game you jump on his head three times defeating the dragon, he disappears and the keys falls down from the heaven into your hand and then the victory song comes on.

Not all doctors are foolish, greedy, and selfish. There are many health care providers have still maintain their integrity and because of that millions of people are healed because of the high quality of integrity that leading doctors and providers have harnessed and delivered to the children of God. That leaves many more millions to struggle to find the answers to question they thought that there was no answers to. May I add; some doctors & providers do maximize their God given talents by giving you the very best advice to help you care for your body faithfully, they are faithful (priceless).

There's not a single birth defect that can come as a genetic inheritance. But many human beings lose their baby's every day. Millions of babies are being born with birth defects and yet we are tolerant of this criminal behavior. Minerals and vitamins could have given before the break down of cells.

They give it to the dogs. Nutrition is by far cheaper & healthier for our countries. God says that they sit and (conspire) presentence) against the children of God. That means in order to keep the ball rolling they must keep coming together against us. The secret is out; people are taking their lives and health back. I believe the medical industry will be more humble and the love will return because money can be a good source but is the root of all evil. People are running a race to see who is going to be the leaders of these countries. They feel like they'll use your ignorance; insurance and money makes no difference as a pathway to make them rich. Beware they have more diseases they call <u>NEW</u> in there stash for the world. There's nothing <u>NEW</u> Under the sun they take them out like a bag of tricks.

Epigenetic is a name given to a process by which you're DNA & your genes require certain nutrients to maximize their genetic potential. What do you have if you don't get the required nutrients?

A glitch (malfunction, fault, abnormally, dilemma, technical hitch like a phrase we use for a computer when it malfunctions. Some doctors will say "Oh well, it's normal because it's in your family," so that you can be rid (unarmed) of more questions about you and your loved ones' condition. (No more questions). Questions lead you to vital information. If you have the right information you can win a war even if it is in your body.

You won't seek to fix the problem because you think that your problems are normal even though you have symptoms that are life altering causing you not to be conducive (favorable, beneficial & contributing).

But I tell you the truth as God lives and have made us perfect in His sight and deemed us good, the mal nutritional situation you're experiencing is a direct result of the spirit of greed in human being.

It is not normal for you to depend on a machine to live. The adversary has crept in and has caused much havoc in the land, but I say to you he will be thrown into the lake of fire for what he has done, and his workers with him.

In their endeavor to see the sheep slaughtered they find themselves in the pit they dug for us. If they don't repent hell waits. Pastors are preaching to a bunch of sick people. They are sick in their hearts and minds many things are overlooked, many can't make decisions on how to live a healthy and productive life because many are still unarmed. I say to you today arm yourself.

Put on the whole armor of God so that you can stand against the wilds of the devil, we wrestle not against flesh and blood but against principalities, spiritual wickedness in high places (powers of darkness). God said to anyone who comes to God must believe that he is and a rewards them that diligently seek Him. When do we draw the line in the sand?).

Don't waste precious energy being upset with your enemies, vengeance is mine, I will repay says the Lord.

Pray for God to heal you, don't be afraid to asks questions and look in a book and read up on your conditions if a doctor diagnoses you with any disease ask him/her "what is the criteria for this disease?" Write down everything, go home and sit down and have a little chat with your Lord (the one who has complete authority, control, and mastery over you) God may say who told you; you had this or that and you wait for instructions from the Lord.

The problem with most people is that they wait until something goes wrong to seek the Lord. God says OK well I can deal with it; I'll just use this situation to bring them to me. Look up the diagnosis on the internet or in a book because your future is now in your hands. When you've done all to stand; stand therefore knowing that God is on your side.

Do what God says for you to do concerning your body. Jehovah is our God He sent His only begotten son Jesus who is the true Christ into this world the as propitiation for our sins because there was no other way that we could be redeemed. This proves that He really loves you. When we are sick & in pain we ask where is God? Many in their ignorance have turned away from the ways of the Lord unto other gods, (the doctors) which have lead to many illnesses. When you turn away from the Lord your hearing becomes dimmer and dimmer; The Lord says my sheep knows my voice and a strange voice they will not follow. We have to follow God every day. God says ''This evil I have seen under the son a man to whom the Lord Give riches so much that he/she don't even want for their own soul''.

Churches have 5,000 members that won't do nothing but 800 that will pull the load, they'll work in the Kingdom.

SPALMS 24

The earth is the lords and the fullness there of the world and they that dwell in it, he had founded the seas established it on the floods who will ascend into the hill of the Lord? Who will stand in His Holy Place? He that has clean hands and a pure heart; who have not lifted up his soul to vanity nor sworn deceitfully he will receive the blessing from the Lord and righteousness from the God of his salvation. This is the generation that seek Him seek thy face oh Jacob.

Lift up your heads oh you gate and be lifted up you everlasting doors and the King of Glory will come in. Who is the King of glory!? The Lord Strong! And Mighty! The Lord Mighty in Battle. Lift up your heads oh you gates even lift them you everlasting doors and the King of Glory will come in. Who is this King of Glory!? The Lord of Host He is the King of Glory.

Psalms takes us in into Israel's worship life experience, if you are a child of God and you have a relationship with God you should have a strong worship lifestyle it should be solid.

Israel's lifestyle of worship is an example to us to show us what a life of devotion looks like. Yes we sin and often fall short of the glory but, but, but when we get in His presents there is fullness of Joy. God has chosen someone for you to lead you into His presence so that you can have this same experience of worship. Now isn't He good. That is why some of us go to church but that doesn't limit God when you don't, because that's why you went to the base ball game or to that old restaurant you thought you were going for another reason but in up asking Jesus be become you savior. We are becoming a bunch of rich, tongue talking moon walking powerless saint. We have material possessions of every kind stay with God.

Praise God! He gives us gifts so that we can preach teach pray, sing and some of us are teachers, scientist, pilots, lawyers, doctors, gymnast, basketball, baseball, management, office personnel speaking in tongues interpretation of tongues and professors. During the course of the day we do our jobs and some of us are incorporated in God's divine work Soul winning because this is not our home, we don't want to go to heaven by ourselves do we. After we do all of that, your personal day to day walk with the Lord that makes a difference.

We can work and be a lousy person if we don't have that day to day encounter with our Lord during the day and after we clock out. You need to have had more than a normal church experience. Psalms has poetry, prophecy that Jesus would stay on the cross ''my God my God why have you forsaking me?'' The psalm are also prayers we have the psalm of supplication and, prayer ''unto thee oh Lord I lift up my soul oh my God I trust in you, let me not be ashamed let not my enemies triumph over me. Some give praise and adoration where you lift up the name of the Lord and the greatness of God you magnify His name.

'' Great is the Lord and greatly to be praise in the city of our God in the mountain of His Holiness beauty for situation joy of the old earth in Mount Zion on the side of the North the city of the great King. Gratitude ''thy love in kindness is better than life my lips will praise you and thus will I bless you I lift up my hands unto thy name ''as the heart panteth after the water so my soul panteth and longest after you oh Lord there's nothing that can lift you quickly you go the psalms if you are trying to get through from day to day trying to make it overcome depression trying to fight evil psalms very therapeutic you can get off drugs take vitamins and minerals but the Holy Spirit is for your soul and that is missing in millions of people your spirit will cry out for the living God if you cannot understand that your head will hurt because of the stress in your body. If you go to the doctor they will medicate you but if you come to Jesus our blessed savior he will fill you up with His Holy Spirit. David says my cup runs over. The song says come to Jesus my blessed savior His is worthy to be praised. Lay down your burdens at the feet of Jesus and leave them there. The Lord is my light and my salvation; ''who should I fear? The Lord is the strength of my life' whom will I be afraid? When the wicked (some doctors) come upon me to eat up my flesh they stumble and fell though a host encamp against me in this I will be confident.

Think on Him! he is my life my joy the center of my heart blessed is the person that who walks not in the counsel of the ungodly (some doctors) nor stands in the way of sinners nor sit in the set of the scornful but his/her delight is in the law of the Lord and in His law he/she meditates day in night and you will be like a tree planted (rooted) by the rivers of water

(Never be thirsty) seasoned who bring forth fruit in your season whose leaves will not weather and whatever you do will prosper.

24th psalm is the most majestic psalms among the processional psalms, processional because when ever Israel came up to the ark of the covenant to that tabernacle or temple there it was always processional'' coming up a certain way'' it was formal you don't just run in and grab a seat like a stadium there's no glorious entrance no magnificence in our worship.

The processional suggest that your entering in and giving glory and Honor and recognition to someone in a superior position that's why he said make a joyful noise unto the Lord all you lands serve the lord with gladness come before His presents with singing know you that the Lord that He is God it is He that made us not we ourselves, we are His people and the sheep of His pastures.
Enter into His gates thanksgiving and into His courts with praise be thankful unto Him and bless His Holy name. For the Lord is good His mercy is everlasting His truth endures unto all generations. Many people like to sit in ponder the goodness of the lord and esteem Him mildly. Psalms suggest that you must come with a certain kind of radical expression sometimes. You haft to open your mouth and say thank you , thank you , thank you thank you thank you, I don't know about you but the more I praise Him the better I feel! 90% meditation on the word of God & in the presents of God and 10% in public worship when you get to where you're going you should be loaded.
I will bless the Lord at all times His praise will continually be in my mouth , my soul shall make her boast in the Lord and the humble will hear and be glad come magnify the Lord with me and let us exalt His name together. It's cross cultural it has nothing to do with the color of your skin or where you were born, just what God demands He is to be adored from the risen of the sun to the going down of the same. The name of the Lord will be exalted! Glory and honor praise and dominion and power to Jesus! To the King of King and to the Lord! Of Lord!
This is the song that they sang when they brought the ark of the covenant presence of God the nation of Israel when David was just made king over all Israel that's why he danced out of his tunic God finally brought the presence of God into his administration so that

His kingdom could be secure because without Him we can do nothing. It wasn't like that always with David he had a breakdown it happens to the best of us he was a man after Gods own heart a anointed musician and a violent worshiper but he had a break down. David wanted the ark in the presence of Israel but he failed earlier the ark was in Shiloh the Philistines confiscated the ark the enemy knows that he could not beat presence of God.

We need to since His presence the nearness of His support if the presence is absent you feel insecure you can't get a word from God, you can't feel Him the word of God is not sharp in your mine, your seeking for a word and can't get one you ought to feel insecure because He is the way the truth and the life.

He is the one who shows and directs He is the one that has a word for your life and so when His presence is absent it can cause you be unstable you don't feel centered and focused praising is therapeutic the more I praise Him the more a feel alive in Him the more I praise Him I receive benefits from him, the more I lift Him up the more He lifts me up, the more I magnify Him, the more He magnify who I am in Him.

My praise boomerangs it comes right back to me why because I can't beat God given. God is not going to allow you to beat Him out in given I don't haft to figure out my own way He say go this way, go that way, do this, and do that, He says your healed, and not sick. Hah- La- lu-yah! Exalt Him. The Philistines stole the presence out of Shiloh it discomforted the people they took the presents of the Lord we are sick without His presents. They thought they could handle it' that proved not all worship is the same' there two types of people before God people who love God and people who don't love God. If you're going to choose to love choose God because man/women will let you down people and things are seasonal but the Holy Spirit is eternal, Het is the only friend that can't be compromise.

His presents will lift you up, or tare you down. If you love God you're in the right place if you love God His presence will bring benefits if you don't love him His presence will make you uncomfortable it could be disastrous, people who don't love him get antsy they start fidgeting and moving around in their set saying' it don't take all that'. I don't know you might be in the wrong place cause we have come into His house to gather in His name to worship Him forgetting about our self concentrating on Him we didn't come to bow down to Alah we didn't come to give praise to Buddha ''all Hell King Jesus''! They took it and put it into their camp and it cause them much agony they placed it next to their God in the temple of Dagon – Dagon means part man part fish out of stone they went through a series of attack they woke up and found Dagon's hands cut off, head cut off, bowing down before God! He doesn't share his glory with another.

God says I have told you the truth & you refuse to listen. I will tell you again.
Gen 29: God said, behold I have given you every herb baring seed, which is upon the face of all the earth, in every tree in which is the fruit of a tree yielding seed to you it will be for meat. - And to every beast of the earth and to every fowl of the air into everything that creeps upon the earth, where there is life.
"(I have given every green herb for meat)", and it was so. Study for your life and your loved ones also. Do what you can do and let God do the rest. He loves you; you were divinely designed by him. Plead the blood of Jesus all power is in his hand. Pray earnestly with praise and thanks giving.
For some of you who are heavenly minded and no earthy good you say; God is going to heal me and you don't do right by your body.

I heard the word say you ought to present your body a living sacrifice hold and acceptable unto God which is only reasonable. (That's all I require).

Daniel was a leader. He resolved not to defile himself with the King's royal food and wine. Now God had caused the official to show favor to Daniel, but the official spoke to Daniel saying "I am afraid of my lord the king, who has assigned your food and drink. What will he say when he sees you looking worse than the other young men your age?

The king would have my head because of you." Daniel then said to the guard whom the chief official had appointed over Daniel, Hananiah, Mishael and Azariah; please test your servants for ten days: Give us nothing but vegetables to eat and water to drink; Then compare our appearance with that of the young men who eat the royal food, and treat your servants in accordance with what you see.

So he agrees to this and tested them for ten days. At the end of the ten days they looked healthier and better nourished than any of the young men who ate the royal food. So the guard took away their choice food and the wine they were to drink and gave them vegetables instead. To these four young men God gave knowledge and understanding of all kinds of literature and learning. And Daniel could understand visions and dreams of all kinds.

At the end of the time of training he presented them to Nebuchadnezzar. The king talked with them, and he found none equal to Daniel, Hananiah, Mishael, and Azariah; so they entered the king's service. In every matter of wisdom and understanding about which the king questioned them, he found them 10X's better than all the magicians, enchanters in his whole kingdom. And Daniel remained there until the first year of King Cyrus.

And now I decree and declare you will not be in bondage of any kind, and that you will be among many a testimony for the nations a blessed temple and you will live before me says God, for you will dwell in my house where I have set my name and in my name you will do wonders only live up right before me and you will have my perpetual blessings as long as you live upon the earth in Jesus name.

2

COPPER

Copper is a micro mineral; a chemical element with the symbol Cu and atomic number 29. It is a ductile metal with very high thermal and electrical conductivity. Pure copper is soft and malleable; a freshly exposed surface has a reddish-orange shinny color.
Copper has low chemical reactivity. In moist air it slowly forms a greenish surface film called patina; this coating protects the metal from further attack.

The copper bracelet fits many sizes on the wrist, it's good for the body and you'll get both of its affects, the positive size of the copper as well as the magnets.
If you have any energies or arthritis this will help.

The copper bracelets also helps with hair color and healing for the eyes and skin & copper also aids in the formation of bone, Hemoglobin and red blood cells works with zinc & vitamin C to form firmness in skin.
Copper makes protein more available to the body by freeing up the iron healing process and energy production; hair & taste sensitivity, nerves, joints, skin, and connective tissue. Copper improves vitamin C oxidation low and high are found in those that have emotional disorders and rid the body of parasites.

Copper is widely known as a brain stimulant which is why food with a high copper content is called brain food.

In regards to your diet use proportions correctly, too much of one thing can be harmful. Copper helps the body to defend itself it is said the perfect cure for anemia, also help stimulate the immune system.

Essential Minerals for Maintenance & Recovery

- Helps people who suffer with arthritis.
- It helps regulate the rhythm of the heart.
- Flushes the kidneys & gastrointestinal track
- Tonic for the liver , spleen & lymphatic system
- Helps in maintaining digestive health
- Helps absorption of iron
- Stimulates the brain
- Produces melanin contributing to the pigmentation of eyes & hair
- Regulates the working of the thyroid gland
- Help relieves authorities & inflamed joints
- Slows down aging in men & women
- Aid in weight loss in men & women
- Helps combat Anemia
- Helps wounds to heal faster
- Help maintain cardiovascular health

- Copper beats hypotension

I recommend not drinking out of the water bottles and buy a water filter. Also drink from copper cups and pitchers.

Symptoms of Copper Deficiency

1. Allergies
2. Kawasaki Disease
3. liver disease
4. Aneurism
5. Arthritis
6. Dry & Brittle Hair
7. Parasites
8. Edema
9. Parkinson's Disease
10. Reduced Glucose Tolerance
11. Hernias
12. Hypo & Hyper Thyroid
13. Varicose Veins
14. Heart Disease
15. Wrinkled skin in men & women
16. Osteoporoses

Natural Source

- Liver
- Almonds
- Leafy Green Vegetables
- Sea Food
- Spinach
- Kale

Essential Minerals for Maintenance & Recovery

Zinc

Minerals are the most overlooked factor of nutrition, when it should be the first thing to be considered. When you look at a patient and he or she has lost blood we know that they will need iron. How the patent is doing determines how the iron should be given to the person. If a person is having heart problems magnesium is perfect because it works instantly and is suitable for treatment because it is good for the body as a whole. Minerals & nutrition are the most important because when your body breaks down it is then you need them the most.

The fundamental factor of all Nutritional factors is the fact that they are so essential; that means we are dead without them. If the minerals are lacking your body, isn't going to utilize all the other vitamins & nutrients.

Minerals regulate the nervous system. If you are deficient in minerals, disease is the poisonous serpent coming down your path; when the disease strikes it is the same effect as that if you were bitten by it.

Zinc ranks in the top three along with vitamin A and Iron that is responsible for taking care of most diseases and they are many.

Symptoms of Zinc Deficiency

- Immune compromise
- Leaky Gut Syndrome (gut leak protein)
- Food allergy
- Mal absorption (not digesting nutrients well)
- Diarrhea (loose stool)
- Irritable bowel syndrome
- Gas & bloating
  Thinning hair or loosing hair
- Inflammation on skin (acne, eczema, & crisis).
- Protein syntactic

Zinc is responsible for thicker hair in men and women. And helps your body grow adequately and repairing of tissues and organs. Decrease high levels of emotional stress. If you've had a loss in your family, stress on the job, or are going through a situation that is mentally and physically challenging, zinc will help your spine stand strong to support you during the time that your body is under stress.

Athletes are most susceptible, bikers, ball players and marathon runners. If your pregnant or breast feeding women because their eating for two.

Aging women tend to have mile absorption although men can have the same experience. (They may not absorb zinc well).

Essential Minerals for Maintenance & Recovery

Iron

Iron is required to make hemoglobin red blood cells act as a vehicle to transport oxygen and nourishments to the bones & tissues. Anemia is affiliated with blood disorder

Anemia Symptoms

Excessive Fatigue
- Decreased appetite
- Rapid heart Rate Shortness of Breath

- Hair Loss
- Cold Hands & Feet
- Sore Tongue
- Easy Bruising
- Brittle Nails
- Dizziness

Low enough can produce a constellation of Symptoms Not anemia but immune system is weak (sick& tired).

Natural **Sources**

Beans
- Spinach
- Pumpkin Seeds
- Liver
- Cuttle fish
- Oysters
- Mollusks

Essential Minerals for Maintenance & Recovery

Magnesium

There's a good chance you may have a health condition If you get more Magnesium in your diet it could be gone – for good. Many people are suffering with conditions that if you get magnesium in your diet it will be transferred out for ever.

According to research 80% of Americans are Magnesium deficient. People need to get more magnesium in their diet. If you are already deficient of it, and you got into an accident your body won't be able to make use of it and you would be better off if you are sufficient in it even to the point of saving your own life. If your magnesium is low you can undergo a sudden cardiac rest with no previous symptoms. 50% do not make it in the E.R (heparin & magnesium) is needed to survive the emergency room.

Symptoms

- Headache, relaxing muscles and cellular function
- Muscle cramps most people identify cramps with potassium it can also be true
- Osteoporosis weak muscles & bones get injured easily; magnesium is major for building strong bones take Vitamin C & magnesium together.
- Diabetes or imbalanced blood sugar
- High Blood pressure (magnesium is one of the

best natural remedy for lowering or balancing blood pressure

- Insomnia not being able to sleep at night/ waking on constant bases -take at dinner or before bedtime.
- Anxiety & depression magnesium has been shown to help calm the body muscles improve more
- Vital for overall mood swings
- Muscle pain
- Migraine head aches

Essential Vitamins for Maintenance & Recovery

3

Vitamin A

Vitamin A Rank in the top three along with Iron & zinc that is responsible for taking care of a lot of diseases. If you are deficient in these you can reap the consequences of being found blind, dumb, and lame.

- Measles
- Leukemia
- Crones Disease
- Liver
- Dandruff
- Taste buds
- Kidney Stones
- Difficult Identifying Blue & yellow aging tissues formation digestion genital organs

Natural Sources

- Eggs
- Fish
- Butter
- Beef
- Liver
- Cream
- Green Vegetables
- Carrots
- Oranges

Type 1 & Type 11 Diabetes

4

- **Blue Berries**
- Great antioxidant dietary fiber
- Vitamin C Falconoid
- Immune Boosting System
- Lower Cholesterol
- I improves glucose control
- Improve insulin sensitivity
- Lowers risk of heart disease

Cranberries
- Disease fighting antioxidant
- Vitamin C
- Prevents Urinary Tract Infections
- Protects against Breast Cancer & Prostate Cancer
- Protects against Heart Disease
- Anti inflammatory
- Lower Cold and Flu Frequency
- Decrease risk of Periodontal Disease

Apples

- Soluble Fiber
- Slows Carbohydrates
- Digestion
- Reduces Glucose
- Stimulates Pancreas
- Decreases risk of Asthma
- Decreases risk of heart disease

Melon

- Watermelon
- High in Vitamin C, A & B
- Protects against cancer
- High in beta carotene
- Lower Blood Pressure
- Improves insulin sensitivity

Honey Dew

- High in Vitamin C
- Source of Potassium
- Improves/ maintains blood Pressure

Rock Melon

- High in potassium
- Antioxidant Beta Carotene
- Fiber
- Vitamin C
- Foliate
- Niacin
- Decrease risk of heart disease
- Promote lung health
- Anti age
- Related macular degeneration

Raspberries

- Fiber
- High in Vitamin C
- Antioxidant for bone & skin health
- Anti cancer activity
- Heart disease Prevention
- Protection against macular degeneration

Red Grapefruit

- Rich in Vitamin C
- Lower LDL Cholesterol
- Lowers triglycerides
- High in antioxidants activity
- Reduces risk of Prostate cancer
- Reduces risk of kidney stones
- Protects against colon cancer
- Boost liver enzymes
- Repair DNA
- Inhabits tumor formation

Tomatoes

- Vitamin C
- Potassium

- Antioxidant Riboflavin
- Chromium
- Helps protect against prostate, Clitoral,
- breast, endometrial, lung &pancreatic cancers
- Reduce heart disease Anti- Inflammation
- protection Reduce blood- clotting tendencies
- Reduce frequency of migraine attacks
- Keep blood Sugar Levels under control

Asparagus

- **Fiber**
- High in Vitamin B foliate Vitamin C
- Antioxidant glutathione
- Boost immune System
- Promote Lung health by Protections against Viruses
- Cardiovascular Benefits
- Helps digestion
- Regulates blood Sugar levels

Carrots

- Fiber
- Vitamin A
- Beta Carotene
- Protects night Vision
- Promotes Lung Health

Broccoli

- More Vitamin C than an Orange
- Wound healing
- Fiber
- Antioxidant beta carotene
- Vitamin A
- Promotes healthy Vision, teeth, bone, and skin Antioxidant
- Anti cancer nutrients

Red Onions

- High in antioxidant power
- Foliate for heart health
- Anti inflammatory
- Can increase bone density
- Benefit to connective tissue

Spinach

- Vitamin B 2 & 6
- Foliate
- Copper
- Calcium
- Magnesium
- Potassium Zinc
- Fiber
- Anti cancer agent
- Anti inflammatory agent
- Agent
- Antioxidant beta carotene
- Protects cells from free radicals
- Prevention of eye problems
- Age related macular degeneration
- Bone supportive nutrient

Fish

- Omega 3
- Can lower triglycerides
  Reduce inflammation
- Better cell function improved communication
- between cells and brain
- Lower blood pressure
- Reduce risk of blood clots
- Cardiovascular protection
- Decrease risk of depression
- Decrease risk of hostility the young
- Decrease risk of cognitive decline in the elderly
- Joint protection
- Decrease of eye related problems

Pineapple

- Constipation and irregular bowel movement
- Rich in fiber
- Morning sickness, motion sickness& nausea
- Bronchitis, diphtheria and chest congestion
- Vitamin C an enzyme called (Bromelain), Surgery and healing wounds, sinusitis, joint & authorities
- Which is known to dissolve loosen up mucus
- Rid of intestinal warms
- Keeps intestines and kidneys clean
- Effective in flushing toxins from the body
- Rich Manganese

Soy

- Highest in Protein
- Niacin
- Foliate

Zinc
- Potassium
- Iron
- Omega 3
- Lowers cholesterol
- Heart health
- Wound Healing
- Lowers blood pressure Water balance
- between cells and body fluids

- Protects menopausal women's bones
- Stabilize blood sugar levels
- Lower risk of diabetes
- Protects against kidney & heart disease related to diabetes
- Lessen chronic inflammation
- Promote gastrointestinal health

Yogurt

- Calcium
- Promotes healthy bones, teeth, muscles & blood vessels
- Vitamin B2 Riboflavin
- Protein
- Zinc
- Aids in immune function
- Helps wounds heal
- Helps digestive system
- Improves cholesterol
- Improves immunity

Flax Seed

- Offers benefits as Omega 3 found in fish
- Lowers triglycerides
- Reduces inflammation
- Decreases the risk of heart disease
- Prevent and control high blood pressure
- High in soluble and insoluble fiber

- Antioxidants
- Protects bone health
- Reduces prostate cancer growth
- Helps ovulation
- Protects post menopausal women from heart disease
- Reduces hot flashes by 60%
- Lowers the risk of dry eye syndrome

Nuts

- Protein
- Fiber
- Vitamin E
- Monounsaturated fat
- Lowers LDL Cholesterol

Beans

- High in Fiber
- Foliate
- Iron
- Magnesium
- Potassium lower risk of heart attack

Oatmeal

- Lowers Cholesterol
- Improves blood pressure
- Stabilizes blood glucose
- Slows digestion

- Antioxidants
- Vitamin E
- Vitamin B
- Magnesium
- Potassium

High Blood Pressure

5

High blood pressure is not contagious or genetic; it's a simple mineral deficiency disease. It can affect anyone and has now spread to our young people of every color and kind. That means it does not discriminate. If you supplement you won't get it.

If you have it, than supplement and it will go away. High blood pressure will then be a memory, and the trial will be something to praise God for. H.B.P medicine lowers the pressure putting you into the dangers of heart attack because the medication lowers you magnesium if your magnesium gets low enough you've compromised your own life as you go into cardiac arrest.

If your thinking well the doctors gave the pills to me, and I ate "just like Adam" Adam died don't let anyone take control your life & health God gave that to you; "you are in control".

The cause of high blood pressure is drugs like **Motrin**, **Ibuprofen**, & the physicians #1 choice **Tylenol**, Are among the top things the devil uses to lead many sheep to the slaughter.

Cure For High Blood Pressure

- **Apples** (**Red & Green**) they have
- Fiber Chlorophyll
- Vitamin C
- Lintel, Elegize acid, Esporta and Quarantine

- Their properties boost the immune system, protect you from cancer, reduce high blood pressure, cholesterol, and lower the risk of prostate cancer.

Celery

- Spleen
- Stomach
- Liver

Relax muscles in and around the arteries making room for blood to flow lowering the pressure.

Cucumber
- Cucumbers are high in
- potassium,
- magnesium &
- fiber
- vitamins A,C,K
- foliate,
- chaffier acid
- Silica,
- Ginger great substitute for salt

- **Kale**

  - Copper
  - Potassium
  - Iron
  - Manganese
  - Phosphorus
  - Vitamins A, C & K
  - Sulfur Python nutrients

Healing for High Blood Pressure

2- Apples

4- Celery

1- Cucumber

1- Ginger (thumb)

6- Kale

Squeeze ½ Lemons

Your Pressure should get normal fast

(Organic fruits& vegetables would be a better choice for healing)

Natural Sources

- Pumpkin Seeds
- Ousters
- Grass Feed Beef
- Sprouted nuts & Seeds
- Flax Seeds
- Almonds
- Peas
- Probiotic
- Keefer
- Sauer kraut

Sauer kraut helps aid in helping to absorb zinc.
Sometimes you have to prepare your body to absorb minerals.

Teeth Health Wheat Grass Benefit

6

Wheat grass has a rich source of enzymes all of our muscle cells and bones are run by enzymes from the time we are born until we die enzymes are responsible for all of our chemical reactions that takes place in the body.

- Loaded with Chlorophyll
- Chlorophyll is an antibacterial
- It stops unfriendly bacteria
- Healing for mouth cancers
- Mouth Oder
- Strep Throat
- Wounds and Herpes soars inside of your mouth
- Chronic Sinusitis
- Nasal problems
- Ear infections
- Ulcers
- Poisons from the gums
- Tooth ache (hold on tooth 5 minutes).

Fillings have tons of poisons. Wheat grass is cheaper, safer, 10X's better than tooth paste. Do you read your tooth paste where it says "(DO NOT SWALLOW)? They put the warning under the directions instead of where it actually belongs in the Warning category. Was that deliberately done so you can over look the fact (true meaning)?

Another meaning for warning is to keep out stay away or how about this one hazard or what about this one dangerous.

Why would you purchase a tooth paste if you see that Warning? The minute your child puts that in his/her mouth they are going to swallow it! Oh! I know it's because of that cool looking commercial you saw on television, and a picture of the lady with the big smile and white sparkling teeth on a bill board and it's very popular on the radio (probably so). Cue the disappointed shaking of the head. If you swallow chlorophyll from wheat grass, your body you feels good because is oxygenates your body. Tissues in your mouth absorb everything.

Chlorophyll is good for your throat, heart, liver, lung & kidneys (preachers, prayer warriors, teachers, professors, and speakers those that are in a profession where you have to repeat speeches or lecture perpetually day after day months after month and year after year this is for you.

Ear Health

7

Hearing loss affects over 36 million adults, or approximately 20% of the adult U.S population the prevalence of hearing loss is raising rapidly because of aging, noise and various health reasons.

The discovery of the formation of free radicals in the inner ear is a key factor in hearing loss. Antioxidants play a role in prevention and therapeutic role.

Experiments have shown a therapeutic effect of antioxidant B- carotene (metabolized to Vitamin A in vivo) and Vitamin C & E on hearing loss & Magnesium is known to reduce noise. Thus B- carotene & Vitamin C & E and Magnesium estimated from both food and dietary supplements, reduce risk of hearing loss and their joint effects in a well defined general U.S population.

National Health and Nutrition Examination 2001-2004

How to Cure an Ear Infection

1. Garlic oil

2. Tea Tree Oil, rub on the outside of the ear around the back

The Cholesterol Hoax
8

Blood ranges from 250-350. They never had organic grown broccoli they are not getting cardiovascular disease. Autopsies show that every animal & human being that dies of natural causes dies of a nutritional deficiency disease. If cholesterol and saturated fat and animal fat were the cause of clogged arteries osteoporosis then it would be the bob cats, foxes and wolves, lions & bears that would have clogged arteries because they are the meat eaters. They eat red meat and fat, the animals that get osteoporosis are the sheep and goats despite the fact they eat grass, grain and hay. Herbivores get osteoporosis and all the carnivores don't (osteoporosis is not caused by elevated blood cholesterol and triglycerides.

Cholesterol is a steroid a raw material that our bodies make it an essential nutrient we must consume it through dairy or otherwise. Male hormone testosterone female hormone estrogen and progesterone they are made up cholesterol the basic raw material that steroid harmonies are made from. Vitamin D, Cholesterol.

L.D.L gets damaged by free radicals eating French fries, fried chicken, fried fish, croutons. It damages the good cholesterol and converts it into the bad cholesterol otherwise cholesterol is cholesterol. We have to keep taking in cholesterol to meet our needs. We also need antioxidants if you can't make them we get these horrible collections of disabling diseases many are life threatening.

There are over 25 diseases that have been created in the last 50 years because physicians have instructed & demanded that their patients give up cholesterol get it out of their diet as a result 25 new diseases seizures disorders to demisters. Alzheimer's disease rank number four in adults over 65. Metamucil is good for cholesterol.

75% of our brain weight is a fatty insulation material melon is about 100% cholesterol you only make about 10% of you daily the other 90% must come from your food- red meat dairy butter & chicken skin you're going to be one that would be a high candidate for Alzheimer's disease.

14 million will die of Alzheimer's disease. Alzheimer's is not a genetic disease.

Alzheimer's was eliminated in animals more than 60 years ago with supplement of cholesterol omega 3 & 6 fatty acids high doses of antioxidants. Large doses of vitamin E & C within months they were able to function again.

Cholesterol is a major factor for fertility. Many people have trouble with impatience because they don't have enough cholesterol to make sex hormones. Men stop being interested in chasing their wives around the kitchen. Is he on a low cholesterol diet? Are you on a high cryohydrate diet? If so you are in danger of getting cataracts and heart disease.

How can people smoke & drink alcohol have clear arteries they were taking in antioxidants fresh vegetables fertilized with wood ashes minerals were over from car denary ashes? We don't have high quality fuel to fill up our bodies.

Kidneys

9

Your kidneys are a blood filter vital for survival Diabetes is a common form of kidney disease. Pharmaceutical & recreational Drugs are a common cause of blood poisoning causing this unwanted circumstance. More than 18 Million people living with kidney disease. The kidneys are your Michaels yes your internal angels they watch over you from the inside out. Your kidneys are working 24-7. They warn, help and protect you. Your kidneys are asking you today to help them save you and not put them into shock by taking drugs, eating unhealthy and getting plenty of rest and plenty of water.

They are tired of suffering from dehydration. When your kidneys need water they will pull water from other parts of the body for example: the brain causing you to be unusually tired, from the colon causing you to have constipation. 95% of people who have kidney failure there's nothing wrong with the kidneys. Due to drugs of all kinds', alcohol, sugar, caffeine, Energy drinks, holding urine and Sodas.

Prevent the process of carrying the dirty blood out of your system. Too much junk (gunk) they get clogged instead of the doctors unclogging them and flushing them they say you have to go on dialysis or worse you need a kidney transplant and what's even worse in your ignorance you're on the table, they take your kidney out and low and behold your kidney looks just fine. Would you throw away a kidney that's good? No '' what are they doing with good kidneys? Are they selling them to the highest bidder?

Symptoms

- Dry eyes & skin
- Weak vessels
- Edema In Legs
- Heel Spurs
- Head Ache
- Lower Back Pain

Natural Sources (Food that cleanse the kidneys)

- Grapes
- Cranberries
- Dandelion
- Cuann Pepper
- Thermal
- Cucumber
- Kidney Beans
- Sprouted Nuts
- Lemon
- Pink Grape Fruit
- Garlic
- Ginger
- Massage

Finding Good Ground

10

Your consciousness is your awareness of yourself and your environment. Some chemicals known as psychoactive drugs alter your consciousness. Drugs affect your perceptions. There are three kinds of <u>Depressants, stimulants</u> and <u>haloclines.</u> Depressants lower your body's functions and activity. For example your heart rate and reaction time has a negative impact on memory and learning process. All are negatively altering weapons.

Ability is the name of the drugs with most sales in 2013 it is an antipsychotic 6.4 billion dollars. Drugs are big business the market has grown into a giant maybe the Philistines in real time ;-) common side effects of drugs are dizziness, nausea, vomiting, and stomach upset. Just in case someone reads this book and has a thought should I continue or stop and make a u turn, mind if I interject and give you this thought. When you love God you care about the things of God.

The root and greater concern psychoactive illnesses brain chemistry are on the rise. What is causing people to go out of their minds? Drugs, fat free diets, not enough raw materials for the singular nerves system to function the way God intended it to be.

What can we do to optimize this? The soil is mineral deficit therefore our bodies are mineral deficit. Agriculture methods have removed the bacteria that are in the soil, the bacteria are in the soil digest the minerals that are in the soil, the plants suck up the digestive minerals and then we eat the plant.

Bacteria are not there to digest the minerals and the plant is mineral deficient the plant is weak, our nutritional food is weak. The farmer have to use pesticides to kill or detour bugs because they don't want to lose the crop, so it's a harsh cycle more and more pesticides, weaker food and it gets perpetually worse never coming up from the grave. Instead of doing it God's way they are rebellious and all of us are still being affected by this unethical behavior.

Winning the War on Your Body

11

More people get lung cancer from frying food than people who smoke. You can reduce the risk of breast cancer by 462 % by cooking your food medium rare rather than well done when you burn the flesh of the animal it develops a life destroying chemicals. Selenium reduces the risk of breast cancer by 82%. Cancer can be prevented, reversed and be stopped. Study shows that there are substances that are in the shark cartel edge that shut off the blood supply to the tumors. Cancer dies when they can't get food and oxygen. Cancer is not genetic doesn't matter if your grandmother died from it and then your mom died from it, you don't have to die from it, you can do the right thing for your body and prevent yourself from getting it.
If anyone dies from prostate cancer it's because the treatment.
- No fried foods
- No Sugar
- No Gluten
- No Deli slices (nitrates & nitrites)
- Cook foods medium rare

Natural Sources

- Liver
- REISHI Mushrooms (the mushroom of immortality)

Mushroomsmatricks.com you can buy mushrooms
Reishi is viable treatment for cancer common colds & flu cardiovascular health.

Mushrooms they have the ability to boost your immune system by 300 % Hoko, Tocki mushrooms limit tumor growth, limit cancer growth even reverse it. These mushrooms kill bad bacteria and viruses even more powerful together for a more powerful effect. Mytocki mushrooms Bunapiai mushrooms they also help our thyroids. **Lion's Mane:** – tonic for the nerves system if you tend to get anxiety high stress put in juice or smoothie.

CORDYCEPS- it comes from the mountains of Tibet it known to fueling Olympians more vitality more strength and skin health.

Become friends with your body, it's impossible to tell people to do the same thing for their bodies and you receive 100% accurate result with few exceptions. People are wondering, "What is the combination to a happy, successful, and healthy lifestyle?"

'A changed mind', we have to empty what we've grown to know. Focus on whole body health instead on dieting.

We have been told so many lies about what our health diet is and have found no real peace and happiness in their remedies. The first thing you need to do is love yourself. Many will reply well I do. Love is what you do not what you feel. You've been doing the wrong things but feeling good while doing it. Paul says everything is expedient, but not all things are profitable. That means you can do whatever you want; ''Question is "where is its profit"?

What does it look like? Bible says you will know the tree by the fruit it bears. That means whatever you are doing to your body will show up in your body. Sometimes the doctors will give you something that's not good for your body. Your body is still your responsibility, how to care for it is still up to you. That means you have to take the time and pray and read.

If you cannot read find someone who can because if you don't that little problem you have can turn into a very big problem with you just listening to the wrong advice. If you keep a healthy repetition your body will recalibrate itself your cells automatically communicate with one another. Your red blood cell will send oxygen to the body and it will be refreshed and rejuvenated and start to work for you. One thing people need to know, if your are on any prescription drugs it should be for a very short time any prescription drug or any other drug will hold back your body from responding the way it should. Many drugs contribute to obesity. If the doctor says you have to take drugs for a long period of time I would look into that because that shouldn't be so.
Sometimes your results are not fast however you don't need a magic ball for an overnight experience. Feel confident that as you're making healthy choices consistently you will reach your goal of ideal health and weight. Give your body what it needs and it will give you what you need. When we love our bodies and treat it well it's going to treat us well, let go of the guilt and the thoughts that lead to depression you want to be lifted mentally- physically and be emotionally stable.
Decisions- decide how I make the right decision for me health wise. Some people have chosen to be a vegetarian or vegan trail blazer, no meat, only fruits and vegetables. Some don't eat dairy and some do. The only problem I have with those choices many are no better off because they don't supplement with vitamins and minerals. They can still acquire some diseases because no matter how much fruits and vegetables you eat more vitamins and nutrients and minerals are simply necessary because the food does not have it all.

How to Naturally Heal Low Stomach Acid

12

- Apple cider vinegar before meal
- Bitters
- Digestive enzymes
- Pep son- hydro caloric acid

Manuka honey –natural antibiotic - keep in medicine cabinet strong antibiotic component to heal cuts or wound wrap it up superior food rich brown -where it differs from your normal table honey this is antifungal- antiviral- antiseptic qualities it can be used internally for minor burns, sores, reflux, heartburn ulcers, and bites. Manuka honey is known to boost energy levels heal minor wounds, infections wounds heal more quickly and a lot less scarring. There's different kinds of Brands you're looking for the brand with label -(UMF on it) unique Manuka factor also associated with a number starting with 10 enriches is the lowest you can get up to the maximum of 24 it tells you how high quality antibacterial that honey does have. If you purchase a UMF 24 you know that you're packing an immense amount of antibacterial properties. New Zealand or Australia it's not affected by heated or the light.

One tea spoon a day or a smoothie, tea, anti aging properties. Balance your gut, helicobacter pylori is a bacterium that develops in your gut it is the trigger that create stomach ulcers. People who eat rich foods need Manuka honey also Manuka is excellent for throat health with lemon and ginger. Manuka & milk is great for relaxing.

Emotional Healing

13

Why am I this way now?
Sometimes in a positive way and sometimes in a bad way some people are naturally lazy others are spunky you have to put some fire behind the lazy one in order to get them to do what they should. The spunky one you may have to pull their coat tail. Others are planners; they have to put you on a schedule. Thieves they can't depend on themselves, murderers a loss of hope for what is good, temperamental people are unpredictable like a time bomb without warning liable to explode anywhere anytime they either don't understand something or when things don't go their way. Experience creates personality.
Often you will find that you need a tune-up to bring about balance. Having a serious personally & devastation in my life I become out of balance, I become too serious, paralyze to deep it has prevented me from enjoying my life for many years.
Jesus broke the strong holds on my life; it took many years of prayer the laying on of hands renouncing immortal activities I had taken part in willingly to achieve deliverance.
 That's why preachers say he picked me up and turned me around place my feet on solid ground.
When we are mismanaged we tend to think deeper than others, when we have been rejected, and beaten vigorously it can cause in balance in your hormones, overdose of I'll spoken words and negativity, not every person born in a stable home with two loving parents and brothers & sister actually have a genuine love for one another.

Trials come into the family and disfigure what families suppose to look like. That's why it is good for the church to come together in the spirit of unity to pray and support one another. God put us together because not one of us has it all we need each other. The song all I need is King Jesus- I don't need nobody else ultimately yes but people tend to overlook the one He sent to bless you to deliver you to minister to you. You're waiting on King Jesus to do what would have already been done.

Many of us are secretive; you just cover up problems and look hard, instead of looking to get them worked out. We find out years later that the reason we don't have any peace is because we've failed ourselves. And your body is letting you know it. You will start to reap the repercussions of the passiveness.

Things will be gain to start tumbling down right on the top of your head. The relationship with your or parents will be affected, your job, everything you do will just be a mess, and you will be standing around saying I don't know what's happening I'm such a good person. God doesn't like me He shows favor to everybody else.

When you get married at the very beginning you will be in love & the next part is going to hurt real good because instead of getting tuned up for your life you will now bring those problems into your marriage and hears the real kicker it would seem like your spouse loves everyone but you.

You won't be able to say anything or do anything without disagreement. Your stress level starts to rise because your body is saying to you stop. Stop you're killing us. And you'll still saying I'm not the bad guy. Sometimes your little life needs to be picked apart because you were torn apart, when you were torn apart there was nobody there to put you back together again, so you just got up and walked way broken. Many times it leaves you mean, disfigured, emotional, aggressive, uneasy, and bitter seems like the devil is trying to still your mind.

You're having a valley experience. One thing about the valley experience is that everything is supposed to get fixed in the valley, you don't come out of the valley undone it would be like coming out of the room naked (awkward feeling). You don't want to do that! So you want to look your best and not like a lunatic leaving the valley on your way to the mountain top! See when you get to the mountain top you shouldn't look like you've been in the valley because that's your testimony.

1 Peter 5 be well balanced for your adversary the devil Rome about like a roaring lion seeking whom he will devoir that telling us that if we would live a balanced life than theirs no opening to get to us. Excess is a play ground for the devil. We were born in sin shaped in iniquity so it's good if we fall on our faces once in a while to produce humility our lifestyle can give us all kinds of avenues that we didn't have before.

Don't forget that we live in a physical world, it could be any moment your life can be changed; many of us don't like change we like the same old raggedy lifestyle and will defend it violently if necessary.

Many are frustrated because things aren't going the way you want. Sin will have too much advantage on you. Surrender to the lord many people come to God after the fact. You come with side effects and you want to get rid of them very quickly.

Things can be fixed but not undone God will deliver you then use you to lead a nation to freedom. Battle is skill against skill competition not injury not kill that the difference between us and the devil God says his desire is to still kill & to destroy.

But I came to give you life that you may have it more abundantly. In a competition if one gets injured the competition is over the ref calls it you have a rank a ref & rules to protect you, to keep everyone from fatal damage.

Listen I am with you and will keep watch over you with care where ever you go and will bring you back to this land for I will not leave you until I have done all of which I have told you.

Are you discouraged over dreams and hopes and nothing seems to be happening you've got to fight the devil with the word of God "what do you know"? If you think about fighting a Chinese he'll say I know kung fu a type of fighting that if you are hit you can reap great consequences & repercussions. Our battles are spiritual we need to know spiritual war fare. If you don't now spiritual war fare you better know someone who does because the devil can come into to your house and reap havoc of it.

14

Many are feeling the effects of going on with their lives without supplementing. People try in rationalizing asking ''which ones to take? And what is the proper per portion? Take all of the essential **60** minerals, **16** vitamins, **12** amino acids, & **2** fatty acids to heal past progressive problems and eliminate any new ones. 90 to life Company is the only incorporation that has every one of them and in its proper proportions so that you don't have to worry about get too much or too little it's just right. No more feelings of sluggish, memory loss, headaches, fatigue, nervousness and even the feelings of depression. Without them your bodies turn against you because it responds when it's not getting what it needs.

15

No drugs no chemicals needed. By the time young women get to be about 20 and 30 they could be diagnosed with a fibroid tumor one or more they can grow in your womb until they cause problems. Doctor will say if they are not causing a problem they don't bother with them you don't want to wait until they get out of control.

They'll suggest that you let them cut them off but they can grow back set you up so that the only you would be able to deliver your baby is through a cesarean section or have a hysterectomy instead of vaginal birth. Fibroid tumors are caused by a Vitamin & mineral deficiency. Our metabolisms are not all the same. All that sugar and junk food things that you eat it won't show up in your blood when it is drawn junk food feeds the fibroid tumors.

- Exercise vigorously
- Red raspberry tea
- Fruits and vegetables
- Dandelion tea (flush liver out of excess
- estrogen
- No process foods
- Cranberry juice
- Water

Beet Juice

Potent nutritional components the beet juice is for

- lowering blood pressure
- increasing athletic performance
- purifying the blood stream
- improving cardio vascular health
- reducing inflammation in the body

you can eat raw beets (the extracted juice liquid that produces the greatest health When vegetables are juiced that are 10 X's more nutritional rich because their nutrition's compounds are highly concentrated as a result this Burgundy Red juice contains substantial amounts of Antioxidants, naturally occurring nitrates, and iron all super healthy ingredients beets are particularly high in.

Prevent & Restore to health of these & many more

- Aids/HIV, Alzheimer's, Anaphylaxis Anemia
- Authorities' Asthma, Bruise Easily
- Cancer, Cold Cores/Fever Blisters Congenital Heart Disorder, Convention, Diabetes, Stroke
- Drug Addiction, Emphysema, Epilepsy or Seizures,
- Fainting Spells/Dizziness
- Frequent Cough, Diarrhea, Headaches, Genital Herpes
  Glaucoma, Hay Fever, Heart Attract, Heart
- Murmur, Hemophilia, Hepatitis A, B or C High Blood Pressure,
- Hives or Rash, Hypoglycemia
- Kidney Problems, Leukemia, Liver Disease, Low Blood Pressure, Lung Disease, Pain in jaw joints,
- Parathyroid Disease, Psychiatric Problems,
- Radiation Exposure, Weight Loss, Rheumatic Fever
- Rheumatism, Scarlet Fever, Shingles, Sickle Cell Disease
- Sinus Trouble, Spinal Bifida, Stomach intestinal Disease, Stroke, Swelling of Limbs
- Thyroid, Tonsillitis, Tumors or Growths, Ulcers,
- Venereal Disease Yellow Jaundice
- Cleft Palate, psychosomatic Disorder .....

Contact Information

Dr. Shakinah Glory Russell

P.O Box 22246
Treasure Cay Bahamas
DRSHAKINHGLORY@GMAIL.COM

Drshakinahglory.my9oforlife.com

Lord Jesus I'm a sinner I believe you died on the cross for me and rose on the third day. I want you to come into my heart and be my savior
I receive you from this day forward Thank You
Now go to a church and talk to a reliable Pastor tell him/her what you have done and they will take you under their wing in Jesus name.
Don't let anybody take advantage of you, use the common since that God gave you. Sometimes we are venerable and the devil knows that read your word learn your scriptures so you can know the truth that you rely on no man but the Holy Spirit only write me anytime and I will respond quickly as possible be blessed.

www.ingramcontent.com/pod-product-compliance
Lightning Source LLC
Chambersburg PA
CBHW071813170526
45167CB00003B/1293